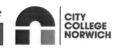

ABC OF ASTHMA

ABC OF ASTHMA

JOHN REES MD FRCP

Senior lecturer and consultant physician, Guy's Hospital Medical School, London

and

JOHN PRICE MD FRCP DCH

Consultant paediatrician, King's College Hospital, London

Articles published in the
British Medical Journal

Published by the British Medical Association
Tavistock Square, London WC1H 9JR

First edition 1984
Second impression 1985
Second edition 1989

British Library Cataloguing in Publication Data

Rees, John, 1949–
    ABC of asthma.—2nd ed.
    1. Man. Bronchi. Asthma
    I. Title II. Price, John, 1944– III. British
medical journal
    616.2'38

ISBN 0–7279–0226–1

Typeset by Eta Services (Typesetters) Ltd, Beccles, Suffolk
Printed in Great Britain at the University Press, Cambridge

Contents

The illustration on the back cover is reproduced by kind permission of the Wellcome Institute Library, London.

INTRODUCTION

There have been a number of changes in the management of asthma since 1984, when the first edition of *ABC of Asthma* was published. But there is also evidence from several countries that the disease is gradually becoming more frequent and more severe.

In most countries the asthma mortality rate continues to be unnecessarily high. Investigations of deaths from asthma have revealed that in many cases the severity of the disease had not been recognised. Many deaths could be prevented if proper use were made of the treatments available. In New Zealand, in the early 1980s, there was a dramatic increase in deaths from asthma; however, these have now declined considerably from the peak rate. As in the case of the 1960s peak in the United Kingdom, the cause of the sudden increase is uncertain.

Morbidity from asthma is still a problem. Studies of airway histology and bronchial reactivity have shown that inflammatory changes in the airway wall remain even when the disease seems relatively quiescent. These investigations have shown that regular treatment and the suppression of persistent inflammation is far more effective than reacting to difficulties as they arise. But to follow such a course we need the understanding and cooperation of patients; we must therefore increase our efforts to educate them.

A few asthmatic patients continue to give great trouble even when all available methods of treatment have been tried. Most patients, however, can be well controlled with current medication without significant side effects. The challenge is to get the right drugs to the patient at the right time. The continuing morbidity and mortality show that we are still failing in this challenge.

J R

DEFINITION AND DIAGNOSIS

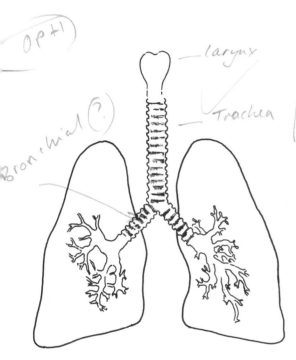

Asthma is characterised by wide variations over short periods in resistance to airflow in intrapulmonary airways.

Asthma is a common condition, yet it continues to be underdiagnosed and undertreated. Asthma is easy to recognise in patients who develop wheezing and airflow obstruction shortly after a specific stimulus, but there is no universally acceptable definition of asthma that includes more chronic illness.

The characteristic feature of asthma is reversibility of airflow obstruction over short periods of time, usually either bronchoconstriction in response to specific stimuli or bronchodilatation in response to treatment.

A commonly used definition of asthma is: a disease characterised by wide variations over short periods of time in resistance to airflow in intrapulmonary airways.

Clinically, the important feature is the recognition of airflow obstruction and the appropriate treatment, rather than the precise diagnostic label used. In children there has been a tendency to use labels such as "wheezy bronchitis," apparently in an attempt to spare the parental anxiety which might be associated with the use of the term "asthma." This avoidance of the term "asthma" is associated with the use of inappropriate treatment—antibiotics instead of bronchodilators and other asthma therapy. The persistence of asthma symptoms is likely to be much more worrying to parents than the use of the word "asthma" accompanied by an adequate explanation. The particular problems of diagnosing asthma in young children will be dealt with in a later chapter.

In the older age group there are difficulties in differentiating asthma from chronic bronchitis and emphysema, diseases associated with smoking. Since few treatments help such patients nobody with evidence of airflow obstruction should be denied an adequate trial of therapy to assess the degree of possible reversibility.

Prevalence

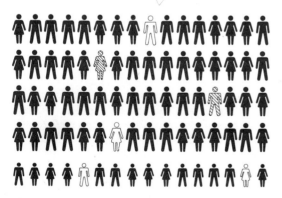

A general practice of 2000 patients will contain over one hundred patients with asthma who have had symptoms or received treatment in the past year; many of those with symptoms may not have had their disease recognised.

The reported prevalence depends on the age of the population studied and the criteria used for the diagnosis. Many of those who do not have symptoms of asthma will have evidence of non-specific irritability of the bronchi if properly tested for airway reactivity. This may mean that they have the potential to develop asthma given the right stimuli.

Ten to 30% of subjects will give a history of wheezing at some time in response to a questionnaire. In many cases, however, the wheezing occurs after a viral infection in otherwise normal subjects: they develop temporary abnormal reactivity of the airways which causes mild transient airway narrowing and wheezing in response to non-specific stimuli. When asthma is diagnosed on the basis of sustained or recurrent symptoms then the prevalence is thought to be around 5% in the United Kingdom and the USA. Some communities have much lower rates, such as Eskimos and North American Indians, while in Australia and New Zealand prevalence is higher. In children in the 7 to 11 year old age group the prevalence is above 10%—commoner than any other significant chronic disease.

The importance of genetic factors is shown by the high rates on the island of Tristan da Cunha, which can be traced back to three asthmatic women among the original settlers. Among children boys are more often affected (by a ratio of around 2:1), but later the sex incidence becomes equal as boys are more likely to show improvement with age.

Definition and diagnosis

Types of asthma

A cough may be the only symptom of asthma, especially in children

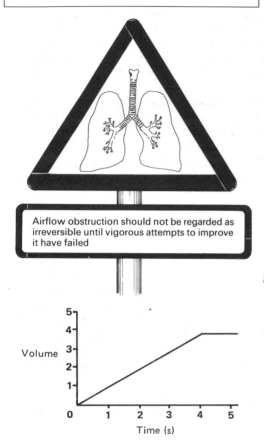

Airflow obstruction should not be regarded as irreversible until vigorous attempts to improve it have failed

A rigid obstruction of a single large airway produces a single wheeze and a fixed flow rate on the spirometry trace (above) or flow–volume loop.

Asthma developing during childhood usually shows considerable spontaneous variability. In young people with asthma there are identifiable factors which provoke wheezing, although patients rarely have a single identifiable extrinsic cause for all their attacks. This "extrinsic" asthma is often associated with other features of atopy such as rhinitis and eczema. When asthma begins in adult life the airflow obstruction is often more persistent and most exacerbations have no obvious stimuli other than respiratory tract infections. This pattern is often labelled "intrinsic" asthma.

Apart from these two broad categories of asthma, there are many who overlap the various forms. Asthma in childhood may well return in adult life after a period of relative freedom. Other important patterns to recognise are those where cough is the predominant or only symptom and those where asthma is associated with occupational exposure.

There are some traps to beware of in the diagnosis of asthma. In children a cough, especially a nocturnal cough, may be the only presenting symptom. This presentation is less common in adults but asthma is always worth considering as the cause of chronic unexplained cough. Airways obstruction may not in fact be present and such patients may not fit the conventional diagnostic criteria of asthma although they show bronchial hyperresponsiveness to non-specific challenge and their symptoms resolve with asthma treatments. In some series 50% of chronic unexplained coughs are eventually diagnosed as asthma. Two other problems in adults are a complaint of tightness in the chest on exertion, which may sound like angina on superficial questioning, and breathlessness at night, which can be confused with the paroxysmal nocturnal dyspnoea of cardiac failure.

The reversible airflow obstruction of asthma needs to be distinguished from the irreversible obstruction of chronic bronchitis and emphysema. It may need vigorous treatment (including a trial of oral corticosteroids) to be sure that the airways obstruction is irreversible, and asthma should not be excluded until such vigorous treatment has failed. Long term treatment regimens can then be planned according to the responses.

Other causes of wheezing, such as obstruction of large airways, occasionally produce problems, most often laryngeal or tracheal narrowing. These may be identified from the single pitch of a wheeze on inspiration and expiration rather than the multiple wheezes of asthma. Appropriate x rays and more sophisticated lung function tests, such as flow volume loops, are needed to find the precise site of the obstruction. In children inhaled foreign bodies should always be suspected as a cause of wheezing, particularly if there is a sudden onset.

Recording airflow obstruction

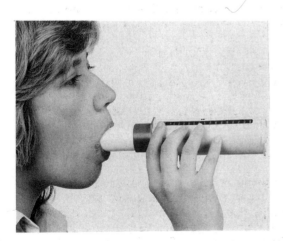

Mini peak flow meters provide a cheap and reliable method of measuring airflow obstruction. Patients can easily use them at home to assess objectively their own control of asthma and response to treatment.

Although acute attacks of asthma occasionally have a sudden, catastrophic onset they are more usually preceded by a gradual deterioration in control, which may not be noticed until it is quite advanced. A minority of patients are unaware of moderate changes in airflow obstruction even when they occur acutely, and these patients are at particular risk of suffering an acute exacerbation without warning. Peak flow recordings entered on simple diary cards allow them to see such trends at a glance, so they can adjust their treatment to prevent acute attacks.

Mini peak flow meters can be obtained for less than £10 and have an important role in educating patients about their asthma. They should be much more widely used and be seen as the equivalent in asthma to routine urine tests in diabetes. Based on their home recordings, people with asthma can develop plans with criteria which stimulate a change in treatment, a visit to the doctor, or an emergency admission to hospital.

Responsiveness to bronchodilators

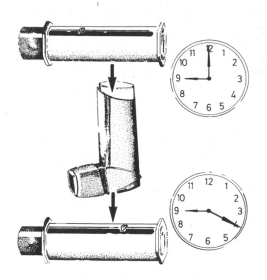

Responses to bronchodilators are easy to assess in the clinic or surgery. Assessing the response can be used to establish a diagnosis of asthma and to determine the most effective bronchodilator. Responsiveness should first be assessed with a selective β_2 stimulant such as salbutamol or terbutaline. This is given as a supervised inhalation of two puffs from a standard metered dose inhaler; this dose can be given freely even to patients with ischaemic heart disease. An increase of 15% in peak flow is generally considered to be significant. If this is not produced by the standard dose the procedure can be repeated after a larger dose of β_2 stimulant or after inhalations of the anticholinergic agent ipratropium bromide. Ipratropium has a slower onset of action than salbutamol and its effect should be assessed at 40–60 minutes rather than 20 minutes after inhalation.

When obstruction is severe and reversibility limited strict measurement criteria may be inappropriate, but any response is worth while, so attention should be paid to subjective responses and the improvement of exercise tolerance or other respiratory function tests.

Decisions about treatment from such single dose studies should be backed up by further objective and subjective measurements during long term treatment.

Diurnal variation

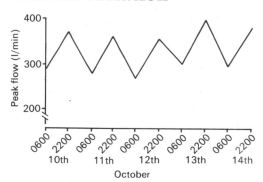

A characteristic feature of asthma is a cyclical variation in the degree of airflow obstruction throughout the day. The lowest peak flow values occur in the morning and the highest values are seen in the afternoon. A peak flow meter should be used to measure peak flow two or three times a day. Asthmatic patients usually show a difference of at least 15% between mean morning and evening values. The cause of this diurnal variation in airway calibre is not clear but its documentation by means of recordings from a peak flow meter made at home is a simple way of confirming the diagnosis of asthma.

People with asthma commonly complain of waking in the night. Deaths from asthma are more likely to occur in the early hours of the morning.

Exercise testing

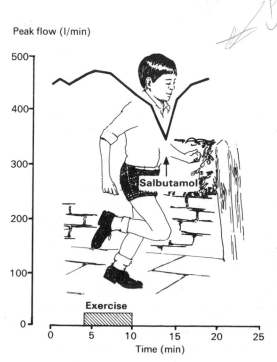

The provocation test most commonly used in the United Kingdom is the exercise test.

Exercise testing is a safe, simple procedure and may be very useful when the diagnosis of asthma is in doubt. When baseline lung function is low testing is unnecessary as reversibility can be shown by bronchodilatation. Exercise testing and recording of diurnal variation are used when the history suggests asthma but lung function is normal when the patient is seen. An exercise test may consist of baseline peak flow measurements then six minutes' vigorous exercise such as running followed by peak flow measurements for 20 minutes afterwards. The exercise is best performed outside since breathing cold dry air intensifies the response. The characteristic asthmatic response is a fall in peak flow of more than 15% several minutes after the end of exercise. Around 90% of asthmatic children will show a positive exercise response. Once peak flow has fallen by 15% the bronchoconstriction should be reversed by inhalation of a bronchodilator. Late reactions are unusual and, unlike allergen challenge, patients do not need to be kept under observation after the initial response has been reversed. Such exercise tests are best avoided if the patient has ischaemic heart disease.

The exercise test relies on change in temperature and osmolality of the airway mucosa. Other tests involving isocapnic hyperventilation, breathing cold, dry air, or osmotic challenge with nebulised distilled water or hypertonic saline provide alternatives. However, they are laboratory based procedures while the simple exercise test for asthma is adaptable to any clinic or surgery.

Definition and diagnosis
Bronchial reactivity

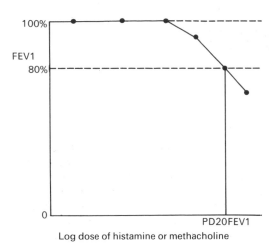

FEV1
100%
80%
0

PD20FEV1

Log dose of histamine or methacholine

Non-asthmatic patients do not respond to exercise; indeed they usually show a small degree of bronchodilatation during the exercise itself. Other forms of non-specific bronchial challenge are inhalation tests with histamine or methacholine. These tests produce a range of responses usually defined in terms of the dose of the challenging agent necessary to produce a drop in FEV1 of at least 20%. Nearly all people with asthma have an abnormally increased responsiveness whereas atopic patients with hayfever but no asthma are an intermediate group. This hyperresponsiveness may well be a basic feature of asthma, reflecting underlying inflammation in the airways. The degree of reactivity reflects the severity of the asthma and can be reduced by avoiding provoking factors or by some prophylactic drugs; but it cannot be reduced by bronchodilators for more than a few hours. The investigation of reactivity is an important epidemiological and research tool. In clinical practice it has little place, except with some difficult diagnostic problems such as persistent cough.

Specific challenge—Challenge with agents to which a patient is thought to be sensitive must be approached with caution. Reactions may be unpredictable: late responses can occur many hours after initial challenges and can lead to poorer asthma control for days or weeks afterwards. These challenges are most often used for investigating occupational asthma but they should be restricted to experienced laboratories.

Skin tests

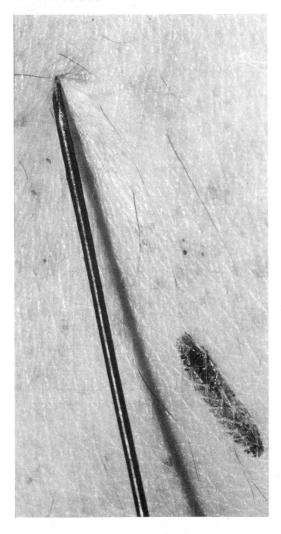

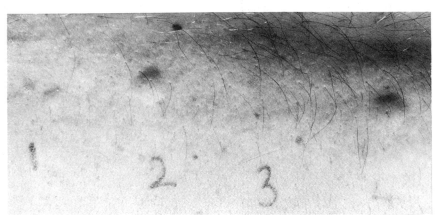

In skin prick tests a small amount of the test substance is introduced into the superficial layers of the epidermis on the tip of a small needle. The test is painless. Most young asthmatics show a range of positive responses to common allergens such as house dust mite, pollens, and animal dander. A wheal occurring after a skin prick test suggests the presence of specific IgE antibody, and the results correlate well with those of in vitro tests for IgE such as the radioallergosorbent test, which is much more expensive.

Positive skin tests do not establish a diagnosis of asthma; they demonstrate only the tendency to produce IgE to common allergens. While more than 20% of the population have positive reactions to skin tests only a quarter of these develop asthma. The importance of allergic factors in asthma is best ascertained from a careful clinical history, taking into account seasonal factors and trials of allergen avoidance. Suspicions may be confirmed by the presence of positive skin test reactions or, on rare occasions, by inhalation challenge.

It would be rare for specific skin tests to be negative when the inhalant allergen tested is important in the patient's asthma. However, the results rely upon the quality of the extract used and will be negative if antihistamines are being taken.

CLINICAL COURSE

Growing out of asthma

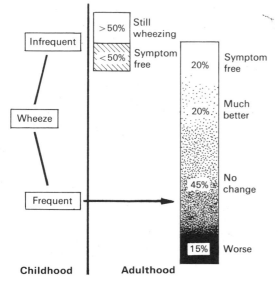

Parents of asthmatic children usually ask whether their child will "grow out of" his asthma. Most wheezy children improve during their teens, but the outlook depends to some extent on the severity of their early disease.

Over half of the children with infrequent wheezing will be free of symptoms by the time they are 21. But of those with frequent, troublesome wheezing only 20% are symptom free at 21, although 20% are substantially better. In 15% asthma becomes more troublesome in early adult years than it ever was in childhood. Even if there is a prolonged remission lasting several years symptoms may return later. After a year free of symptoms airway reactivity remains abnormally high, and a third of these children who have a year's remission will get further symptoms years later.

Asthma is less likely to remit in those with a strong family history of atopy or a personal history of other atopic conditions. More boys than girls are affected by asthma but the girls do less well during adolescence and by adulthood the sex ratio is equal. Chest deformities are uncommon and only occur when there is prolonged severe intractable asthma. Children with asthma usually show normal growth unless they have received long term treatment with systemic corticosteroids, though puberty may be delayed when asthma is severe.

Prognosis in adults

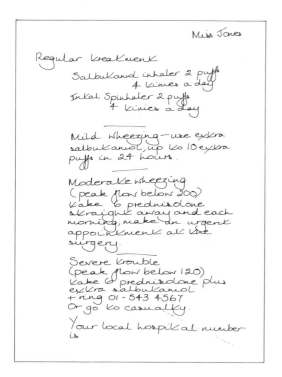

When asthma develops in adults it often shows less spontaneous variation than it does in children. Wheezing is more persistent and there is less association with obvious precipitating factors other than infections. The chances of a sustained remission are also lower than in children. When there are known precipitating factors avoidance of contact with them does decrease bronchial reactivity. Therefore, it is always worth trying to avoid contact with known allergens since this may reduce responses to non-specific agents including cigarette smoke, cold air, and dust.

Smokers with increased bronchial reactivity are particularly at risk of developing chronic irreversible airflow obstruction. This makes it particularly important that asthmatic patients do not smoke.

The reversibility of airways obstruction in asthma is not always maintained throughout life. Those with severe asthma seem most likely to develop irreversible airflow obstruction. It may well be that this progression to irreversibility is related to persistent inflammation in the airway wall, leading to permanent damage. Most chest physicians act on the belief that suitable treatment which reduces inflammation and improves symptoms will reduce the likelihood of long term damage and eventual irreversibility. Without prolonged studies to prove or disprove this contention it seems prudent to follow this practice.

Educating patients about their asthma and the use of treatment is an integral part of management. Patients forget much of what they are told, and information should be backed up by written instructions. It is often helpful to produce these by hand when with the patient. Patients are often confused about the differences between regular prophylactic treatment, such as inhaled corticosteroids or sodium cromoglycate, and quickly effective inhaled bronchodilators used for acute attacks. Regular home use of a mini peak flow meter allows the patient to participate more effectively in the understanding and treatment of his disease.

Clinical course

Genetic factors

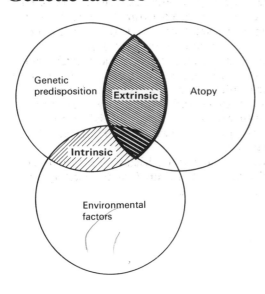

A familial element is well recognised in asthma. But inheritance is not straightforward, and the development of asthma depends on environmental factors acting with the genetic predisposition. Asthma and atopy are commoner in the families of those with extrinsic asthma than in those with intrinsic asthma. Atopy seems to have its own separate inheritance, and the likelihood of asthma is increased when the two genetic predispositions occur together. The movement of racial groups with a low prevalence of asthma from an isolated rural environment to an urban environment increases the prevalence, probably because of their increased exposure to allergens such as house dust mites and fungal spores or to infectious agents and pollution.

The chance of an individual developing asthma by the age of 50 years is increased 20 times if he or she has a first degree relative with asthma. The risk is greater the more severe the asthma in the relative. It was suggested that breast feeding may reduce the risk of a child developing atopic conditions such as asthma because it restricts the exposure to ingested foreign protein in the first few months of life but conflicting studies have been published.

Deaths from asthma

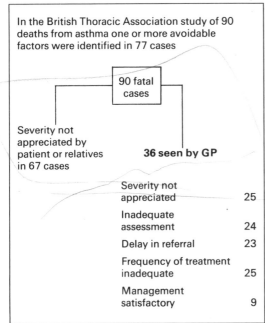

In the British Thoracic Association study of 90 deaths from asthma one or more avoidable factors were identified in 77 cases

90 fatal cases

Severity not appreciated by patient or relatives in 67 cases

36 seen by GP

Severity not appreciated	25
Inadequate assessment	24
Delay in referral	23
Frequency of treatment inadequate	25
Management satisfactory	9

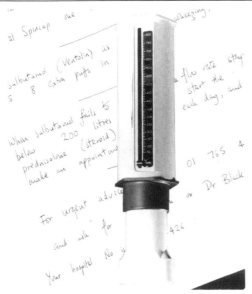

Since the increase in mortality from asthma seen in some countries in the early 1960s there has been concern about the role of treatment in such deaths. Originally the deaths in the 1960s were attributed to cardiac stimulation caused by overuse of inhaled isoprenaline. Many workers have since doubted whether isoprenaline was directly responsible; instead, too great a reliance on its usual efficacy may have delayed appropriate treatment when symptoms worsened. Isoprenaline as a bronchodilator has now been superseded by safer specific β_2 stimulants, and there is nothing to suggest that these inhaled drugs are associated with deaths in asthmatic patients.

The recent increase in mortality from asthma in New Zealand has again aroused controversy, and again the reasons are uncertain. The combination of methylxanthines and β_2 stimulants and the use of home nebulisers have both been blamed, but neither seems to fully explain the problems. The bulge in deaths in New Zealand has largely settled down now and has not been mirrored elsewhere. In the United Kingdom there seems to have been a slight rise in the death rate for asthma. The most reliable statistics come from the 15 to 34 age group where the trend seems to be up. Certainly there is no suggestion of decline and altogether around 2000 deaths from asthma occur in the United Kingdom every year.

In contrast to suggestions that excessive treatment is implicated in such deaths, the British Thoracic Association study showed that treatment in most fatal attacks had been inadequate. Both patients and doctors underestimated the severity of the attacks, and the most important factor was felt to be an apparent reluctance to prescribe corticosteroids for severe asthmatic episodes. Nevertheless, about a quarter of the deaths occurred less than an hour after the start of an exacerbation, and patients showing such rapid deterioration are particularly vulnerable. If patients have shown a swift deterioration in the past they should have suitable treatment, such as steroids and nebulised or injectable bronchodilators, available at home. They and their relatives must be sure of how to obtain immediate further help.

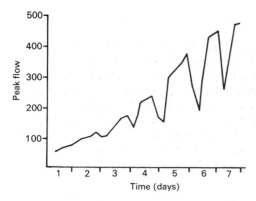

Marked diurnal variation during recovery from a severe attack of asthma.

Several centres have adopted the policy recommended in Edinburgh of maintaining a self admission service for selected asthmatic patients. This avoids delay in admitting patients to hospital and is a logical development to involving patients in the management of their own disease.

Some studies have shown that patients are particularly at risk after they have been discharged from intensive care units to ordinary wards and after discharge from hospital. Problems often occur in the early hours of the morning, at the nadir of the diurnal cycle, and may be related to premature tailing off of the initial intensive therapy on the basis of satisfactory measurements during the day. Adequate supervision and treatment must be maintained through these periods.

Management in hospital has also come under criticism. Treatment and readmission rates are improved when inpatient care is supervised by those with an interest in thoracic medicine.

PRECIPITATING FACTORS

Bronchial reactivity

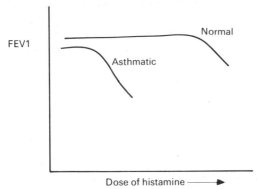

The concept of bronchial reactivity of the airways to specific and non-specific stimuli is discussed on page 4.

The underlying cause of increased bronchial reactivity is uncertain. The sustained reactivity of asthmatic patients has been attributed to imbalance of autonomic control, abnormal immunological and mast cell responses, increased permeability of the airway epithelium, and intrinsic differences in the action of smooth muscle.

Asthmatic airways are usually sensitive to non-specific stimuli such as dust and smoke. Specific responses to agents such as pollen may lead to increased non-specific reactivity for days or even weeks. Upper respiratory viral infections may lead to similar changes and may increase reactivity in non-asthmatic subjects.

Exercise

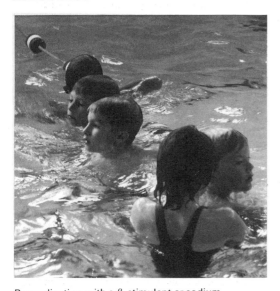

Premedication with a β_2 stimulant or sodium cromoglycate usually allows asthmatic children to participate in sports.

Vigorous exercise produces narrowing of the airways in most asthmatic patients and, as described in the first chapter, can be used as a simple diagnostic test. Asthma during or after exercise is most likely to be a clinical problem in children, where it may interfere with games at school. The type of exercise influences the response; most asthmatics find swimming in warm indoor pools the activity least likely to induce asthma. This clinical observation has now been explained by studies showing the importance of cooling and drying of the airways during hyperventilation and exercise. The effect of exercise can be largely mimicked by breathing cold, dry air; whereas breathing warm, humid air during exercise—as in indoor swimming pools—prevents the asthmatic response.

The best protection against exercise induced asthma is prior inhalation of a β_2 stimulant. Sodium cromoglycate is also usually effective. Such treatment will normally allow a child to take part in games at school. It may be necessary to explain the use of the drugs and the objectives of the treatment to teachers. Exercise itself is unlikely to have any major beneficial effect on asthma, but general fitness and activity should be encouraged. A fit person can perform a given task with less overall ventilation than an unfit one and hence less chance of exercise induced asthma. Asthma is quite compatible with a successful sporting career, as a number of athletes have testified in manufacturers' advertisements.

House dust mites

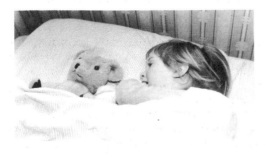

Soft toys may harbour house dust mites in an otherwise clean bedroom.

The house dust mite, *Dermatophagoides pteronyssinus*, provides the material for the commonest positive skin prick test in the United Kingdom. The major allergen is found in the mites' faecal pellets. The mites live off human skin scales and are widely distributed in bedding, carpets, furniture, and soft toys. They thrive best in warm, damp conditions.

If patients move into environments almost free of house dust mites their symptoms may improve. This can be achieved in hospitals but is much more difficult in the home. Nevertheless, regular cleaning of bedrooms and avoiding materials particularly likely to collect dust are worthwhile measures to keep down the antigenic load. More rigorous attempts at complete removal are not justified. House dust mite desensitisation may be of some use in children but not in adults.

Pollen and spores

Pollen or spore production

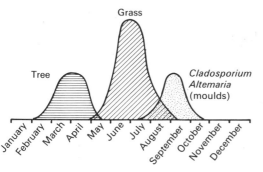

Seasonal asthma, often in association with rhinitis and conjunctivitis, is most usually related to grass pollens, which are commonest during June and July. Less common in the United Kingdom is precipitation by tree pollens, which are produced between February and May, and mould spores from cladosporium and alternaria, which abound in July and August. Complete avoidance of such widespread pollens is impractical.

Hyposensitisation is generally ineffective and unnecessary. Inhaled drugs usually produce perfectly adequate control and are simple to use. The strong placebo effect and allergic reaction to hyposensitisation, and occasional mortality, must also be taken into account in assessing its value.

Some asthmatic patients develop a particular sensitivity to the spores of the fungus *Aspergillus fumigatus*. Allergic bronchopulmonary aspergillosis is associated with marked eosinophilia, rubbery brownish mucus plugs containing fungal hyphae, and with proximal bronchiectasis. Areas of consolidation and collapse may appear on the chest *x* ray and each episode leads to further bronchiectatic damage. The aspergillus skin test is positive and treatment involves long term oral corticosteroids.

Pets

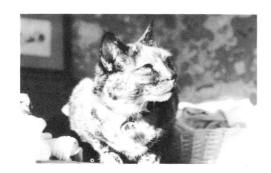

The parents of asthmatic children often worry about household pets. Cats cause the greatest problem, with allergens in saliva, urine, and dander, but most domestic animals can trigger asthma on occasions. Patients who have major problems with their asthma should be advised not to acquire any new pets. Pets already in residence should be kept out of bedrooms and off soft furnishings. If the animal seems to be a major cause of symptoms then a trial separation should occur. Animal dander remains in the house long after the pet is removed so the pet should move out for a month or two; alternatively the patient could move out for a week or two. Unjustified removal of favourite pets without good reason may, however, provoke more problems from emotional upset.

Occupational asthma

Some causes of occupational asthma	
Chemicals	isocyanates
	platinum salts
	epoxy resins
	aluminium
	hair sprays
Vegetable sources	wood dusts
	grains
	coffee beans
	colophony (solders)
	cotton, flax, hemp dust
Enzymes	trypsin
	Bacillus subtilis
Animals	laboratory rodents
	larger mammals
	shellfish
	locusts
	grain weevil, mites
Drug manufacture	penicillins
	piperazine
	salbutamol
	cimetidine

The importance of occupational asthma has been increasingly recognised over the past few years. Some estimates suggest that over 5% of cases of adult asthma have an occupational origin and over 200 precipitating agents have been reported. Asthmatic patients choosing a career should avoid occupations where they are likely to be exposed to large quantities of non-specific stimuli such as dust and cold air.

Occupational asthma is now officially recognised as an industrial disease and subject to compensation. It is defined as "asthma which develops after a variable period of symptomless exposure to a sensitising agent at work." The agents currently recognised for compensation are shown in the box, and this list is being kept under review. Agents such as proteolytic enzymes and laboratory animals are particularly likely to produce problems in atopic subjects, whereas isocyanate asthma is not related to atopic status. In some studies potent agents such as platinum salts have produced asthma in up to half of those exposed.

Increased bronchial reactivity provoked by occupational agents may persist long after removal from exposure. Regular peak flow recordings are once again an important diagnostic tool and usually show a distinct relation to time at work. However, the relationship may not be obvious since the timing of the responses is variable. Reactions may occur soon after arriving at work, be delayed until later in the day, or come on slowly over several days. In some cases even a weekend away from work may not be long enough for lung function to return to normal and absence for a week or two may be necessary. After initial investigation of peak flow patterns at and away from work, further investigation may require specific challenge testing at an experienced laboratory.

Precipitating factors

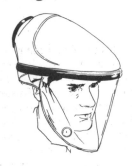

The first approach to management should be to try to adjust the conditions at work that produced the sensitisation. If this is not possible the patient may be able to continue working with a mask to provide filtered air. If these measures fail and simple inhaled treatment is inadequate then a change of job will be necessary. It is advisable to try to obtain, with the patient's consent, the cooperation of any occupational health staff in the firm.

Food allergy

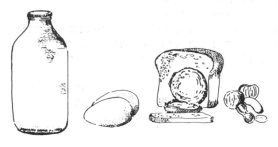

Food intolerance is usually evident from a careful history. Elaborate exclusion diets are rarely justifiable.

Food allergy causes eczema and gastrointestinal upsets more commonly than asthma; exclusion diets have generally been disappointing in asthma. Immediate skin prick tests and radioallergosorbent tests often give negative results. Most serious cases of asthma induced by food intolerance are evident from a carefully taken history, so elaborate diets are not warranted. When there is doubt suspicions can be confirmed by excluding the agent from the diet or by controlled exposure.

Intolerance to food does not always indicate an allergic mechanism. Reactions may be related to pharmacological mediators such as histamine or tyramine in the food. They may be produced by food additives such as the yellow dye tartrazine, which is added to a wide range of foods and medications. When there is a specific allergy to foodstuffs, milk, eggs, nuts, and wheat are most likely to be implicated.

Drug induced asthma

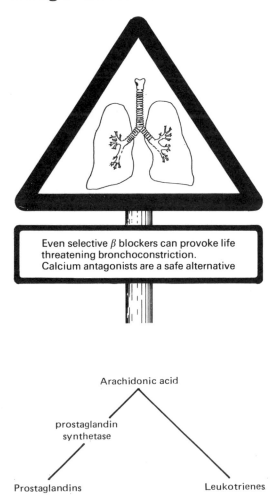

Even selective β blockers can provoke life threatening bronchoconstriction. Calcium antagonists are a safe alternative

Arachidonic acid

prostaglandin synthetase

Prostaglandins   Leukotrienes

Drugs which inhibit prostaglandin synthetase change the balance of prostaglandins and divert arachidonic acid metabolism down the leukotriene pathway.

Two main groups of drugs are responsible for most cases of drug induced asthma: β blocking agents and prostaglandin synthetase inhibitors such as aspirin. β blocking agents usually induce bronchoconstriction when given to asthmatics and this may happen even when they are administered as eye drops. Relatively selective β blockers such as atenolol and metoprolol are less likely to give severe irreversible asthma, but the whole group of β blocking drugs should be avoided in patients known to have asthma. Calcium antagonists such as nifedipine and verapamil are suitable alternatives for the treatment of angina and hypertension and may even be beneficial in blocking exercise induced asthma. When asthma is produced by β blockade very large doses of β stimulants are necessary to reverse it, particularly with non-selective β blockers. Fortunately cardiac side effects of the therapy are not a problem since they are also inhibited by the β blockade.

Salicylates provoke severe airway narrowing in a small group of adults with asthma. Once such a reaction has been noted these patients should avoid contact with aspirin or the newer non-steroidal anti-inflammatory agents, which usually produce the same effects. The mechanism is related to changes in arachidonic acid metabolism. Salicylate sensitivity occurs in more than 15% of adults with asthma and nasal polyps.

Ibuprofen is now available without prescription and produces the same problems. Patients are often unaware of the presence of salicylate in common compound preparations, cold cures, and agents such as Alka-Seltzer. When salicylate sensitivity is suspected the patient should be asked to check carefully the contents of any such medication they may take. When salicylate reactions occur it may be possible to induce tolerance by building up from small oral doses. This should be done in experienced units.

Occasionally drugs used to treat asthma can themselves be responsible for provoking bronchoconstriction. Such paradoxical effects have been described with aminophylline, ipratropium bromide, sodium cromoglycate, and propellants or contaminants from the valve apparatus in metered dose inhalers.

Hypotonic solutions are a potent cause of bronchoconstriction in people with asthma and nebuliser solutions must always be made up with normal saline rather than water.

Emotional factors

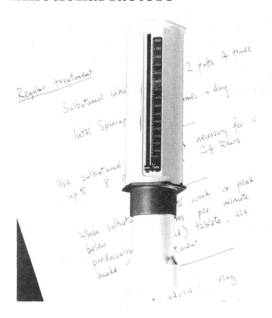

Psychological factors on their own do not produce asthma in subjects without underlying susceptibility. Emotional factors may, however, influence both the bronchoconstrictor responses to various specific and non-specific stimuli and the bronchodilator responses to treatment. Stress and emotional disturbance are just further factors which need to be taken into account in the overall management of asthmatic patients. In children the position is complicated by the emotional responses of the parents. Emotional problems are much more likely to occur when control of asthma is poor, and these problems are best managed by increasing the confidence of patients and relatives with adequate explanation and control of the asthma. It is particularly important that patients know exactly what to do during an acute exacerbation. More specific measures such as hypnotherapy and acupuncture have proved disappointing.

Asthma associated with emotional outbursts such as laughing and crying may be related to the response of the hyperreactive airways to deep inspirations or to inhalation of cold, dry air rather than to the emotion itself.

Manipulative patients may, of course, use a disease such as asthma for their own purposes just as they would use any other chronic disease.

GENERAL MANAGEMENT

Acute asthma: assessment of severity

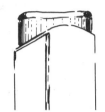

Increasing use of bronchodilator with less effect is a sign of deteriorating control

The speed of onset of acute attacks varies. Some severe episodes come on over minutes with no warning, although more often there is a background of deterioration over days or weeks. This period of deteriorating control of asthma tends to be longer in older patients. If the patient has to use his normal bronchodilator more often than usual but with less effect this is an early indication of trouble. All asthmatic patients should be aware of what to do if they fail to get relief from their usual treatment. The deterioration in control can be detected by regular peak flow monitoring at home. This allows a change of treatment whilst there is a slow decline before severe problems arise.

The most common symptom is breathlessness and this is more often difficulty in inspiration than in expiration. Some patients have a poor appreciation of the changes in the degree of their airflow obstruction and may have few symptoms with moderately severe asthma. They are at particular risk during acute attacks and it is advisable to monitor each patient objectively.

If a patient cannot move from a chair without difficulty it is certainly time to consider admission to hospital. In more severe asthma eating and drinking and even talking may be troublesome. A knowledge of the pattern of previous attacks is helpful as the progress is often similar in subsequent episodes. Patients must be taught to seek help early rather than late in an acute exacerbation. It is easier to step in and pevent deterioration into severe asthma rather than treat a full blown attack. Patients and their families should be confident about the management of exacerbations, both their immediate treatment and hospital admission. A plan of action for crises should always be worked out well in advance.

Examination

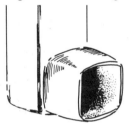

Signs of severe asthma

- Respiratory rate >30/min
- Pulse rate >110/min
- Pulsus paradoxus
- Absence of wheezing
- Peak flow <100 l/min
- Cyanosis
- Hypercapnia

Tachypnoea and inability to speak will be obvious on examination. Cyanosis or confusion caused by hypoxia occurs only in severe asthma and means that admission to hospital and supplemental oxygen are urgently needed. The pulse is a useful guide to severity: a tachycardia of over 110 beats/min is found in severe episodes, although this sign may be less reliable in the elderly, where pulse rates may remain low. Pulses paradoxus (a drop in systolic pressure measured by sphygmomanometer of over 10 mm Hg on inspiration) is not always present in severe asthma but when it is its level correlates well with progress and should be monitored regularly. Any evidence of circulatory embarrassment, such as hypotension, is an indication for hospital admission.

Examination of the chest itself shows a fast respiratory rate, overinflation, and wheezing. In very severe asthma airflow may be too little for an audible wheeze, so a quiet chest in acute asthma is a worrying feature rather than a reassuring one. It may also indicate a pneumothorax. Although pneumothoraces are not common in acute asthma they are difficult to diagnose clinically, and a chest radiograph must be taken if there is any doubt.

In severe attacks the peak flow rate may be unrecordable. Peak flow or forced expiratory volume in one second (FEV1) should be monitored throughout the attack as a reliable, simple guide to the effectiveness of treatment.

In hospital blood gas measurements are also often used to assess progress. Some hypoxia is usual and responds to supplemental oxygen. So long as the patient does not have chronic airflow obstruction there is no need to limit the concentration of supplemental oxygen. The arterial carbon dioxide tension is usually low in acute asthma. Occasionally a high tension is present on admission, but it quickly responds to bronchodilator treatment; this pattern is more common in children. Hypercapnia is, however, an alarming finding in acute asthma, and failure to diminish carbon dioxide retention during the first hour or its development during treatment is an indication that mechanical ventilation must be considered. The final decision on ventilation depends on the overall clinical state of the patient rather than on blood gas measurements.

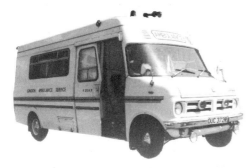

- Problems occur in acute asthma when the patient or doctor fails to recognise the severity of the attack
- Undertreatment is far more dangerous than overtreatment

Where to treat acute asthma

Give initial treatment with bronchodilators, corticosteroids, and oxygen before transfer to hospital.

An acute attack of asthma is very frightening; conceivably transfer to hospital may exacerbate symptoms by producing anxiety, and reassurance that treatment is available to relieve the attack is an important part of management. It is not possible to lay down strict criteria for admission to hospital. The features of severity discussed above should, however, be assessed. Most of the dangers of acute asthma come from a failure to appreciate the severity of an attack and the absence of suitable supervision and treatment to follow up the initial response. Immediate improvement after nebulised salbutamol or intravenous aminophylline may provide false reassurance, being quickly followed by the return of severe asthma. Continued observation is essential.

It may be obvious on first seeing the patient that supplemental oxygen and hospital treatment are necessary. Treatment should be started while this is being arranged. In moderately severe attacks initial treatment should be given and, if the response is inadequate, hospital admission arranged. If the initial response is adequate it may be possible to manage the patient at home if supervision is available. The primary treatment should then be followed up, usually by adequate bronchodilator treatment and corticosteroids, and the response should be assessed by measurement of peak flow.

Deaths from asthma occur when the patient or doctor has failed to appreciate the severity of the attack. When there is any doubt vigorous treatment and admission to hospital are recommended. When treatment is given at home the patient's condition must be assessed regularly and often.

General management of chronic asthma

Obvious precipitating factors should be sought and avoided when practicable. This is possible for specific allergic factors such as animals or foods but is not usually feasible with more widespread allergens such as pollens and dust mites. A common non-specific stimulus is cigarette smoking. Up to a fifth of asthmatics continue to smoke and strenuous efforts must be made to discourage this.

Fortunately most asthmatic patients can have their disease controlled by safe drug treatment with minimal side effects. Education of the patient in understanding his disease and treatment is often helped by home peak flow recording and written explanations of the purpose of treatment. In particular the differences between symptomatic bronchodilator treatment and regular maintenance treatment must be emphasised. It is all too common to find asthmatic patients increasing their dose of inhaled steroid or sodium cromoglycate when an acute attack develops. Trained nurses may be very helpful in continuing education and supervision.

The decision to use regular treatment will depend on the frequency and severity of symptoms. The general approach to long term treatment has moved towards the earlier use of regular prophylactic treatment. Persistent airway inflammation and increased bronchial reactivity have been recognised even in mild asthma. Regular treatment with β agonists such as

General management

	Morning	Afternoon	Evening	Comments
1	240	300	290	
2	220	290	300	
3	230	295	275	
4	200	260	255	Woke at 3am. Wheezy
5	175	235	230	Woke twice.
6	150	190	160	Started prednisolone 30mg
7	190	190	230	
8	250	280	300	
9	330	340	350	
10				
11				
12				
13				
14				

salbutamol may even increase airway responsiveness. The other groups of bronchodilators, theophyllines and anticholinergics, leave reactivity unchanged. On the other hand regular inhaled steroids decrease reactivity and the same may well be true of sodium cromoglycate and nedocromil sodium. The regular use of prophylactic agents is thought to reduce airway inflammation and this may help to prevent irreversible damage. Mild episodes of wheezing occurring once or twice a month can be controlled with inhaled β stimulants. When attacks are more frequent regular treatment with inhaled steroids or sodium cromoglycate is necessary. Definite diurnal variation on peak flow recordings or nocturnal waking indicates a high degree of reactivity of the airways and the need for vigorous treatment.

When chronic symptoms persist in the face of appropriate inhaled treatment a short course of oral corticosteroids often produces improvement, which may last for many months after the course.

The aims of treatment are to avoid problems from persistent symptoms and to treat acute episodes early and vigorously to prevent deterioration into severe asthmatic attacks. In a variable discase such as asthma where monitoring of the state of the disease at home is comparatively easy, patient education and cooperation are a vital part of management. The patient should know how and when to take each treatment, broadly what each does, and exactly what to do if there is an exacerbation.

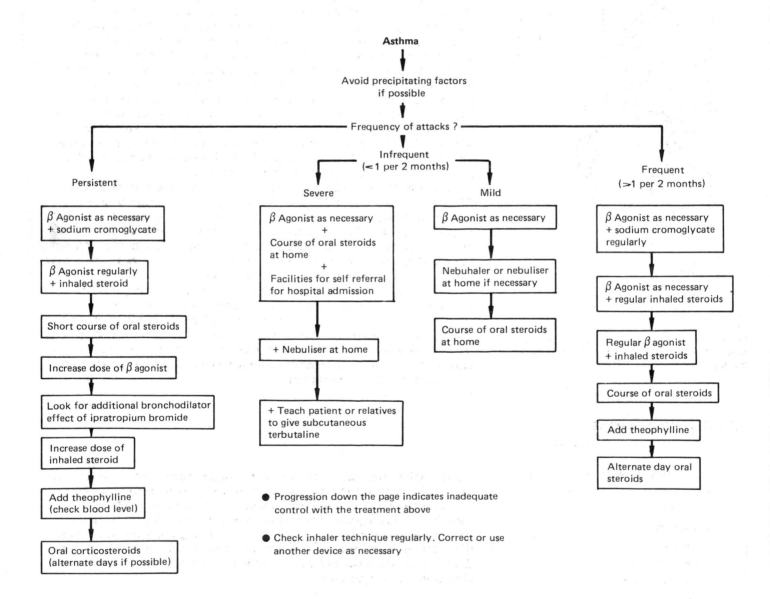

TREATMENT OF ACUTE ASTHMA

β Stimulants

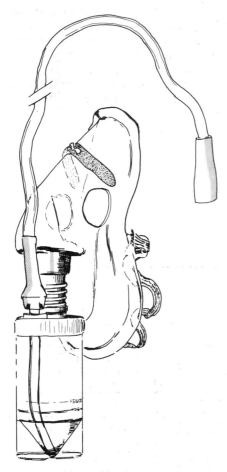

Filling volume, drug dose, driving gas, and flow rate should all be specified when prescribing nebuliser therapy.

Adrenaline has been used in acute asthma for 80 years. The specific β_2 stimulants such as salbutamol, terbutaline, and fenoterol have replaced the earlier non-selective preparations, and within this group there are no great differences in practice.

In acute asthma metered dose inhalers often lose their effectiveness. This is largely because of difficulties in the delivery of drugs to the airways, and an alternative method of administration is necessary—usually by nebuliser or intravenously. An alternative to the nebuliser is the globe spacer (nebuhaler or volumatic). Like the nebuliser it has the advantage of removing the need to coordinate inhaler actuation and breathing. Since there is little or no difference in the effectiveness of nebulised or intravenously administered drugs nebulisation is generally preferrable. Many general practitioners find it useful to have nebulisers available for acute asthma attacks. Theoretically β stimulants are best given using oxygen to drive the nebuliser, as bronchodilator treatment for asthma may occasionally be associated with a worsening of hypoxia. Domiciliary oxygen sets do not provide a sufficient flow to run standard nebulisers efficiently, and therefore nebulisers at home are usually driven by air. It is advisable, however, to have an oxygen cylinder available to treat the hypoxia of acute asthma, even if the nebuliser is driven by air at the same time. There is no real advantage in nebulisation with a machine capable of producing intermittent positive airway pressure.

For adults the initial dose should be 5 mg salbutamol or its equivalent. This should be halved if the patient is known to have ischaemic heart disease. It is essential to continue with the intensive therapy after the first response. Many of the problems in acute asthma arise because the doctor or patient becomes complacent after the initial improvement with inhaled bronchodilators. In severe attacks the nebulisation or bronchodilation may have to be repeated up to every 30 to 60 minutes.

If nebulised drugs are not effective then parenteral therapy must be considered: either β adrenoceptor stimulants by intravenous or subcutaneous injection or intravenous aminophylline. Salbutamol, for instance, can be given as a single injection of 250 µg intravenously or 500 µg subcutaneously or as an infusion of 5–15 µg/min. The adverse side effects of tachycardia and tremor are much commoner after intravenous injection than after nebulisation.

Methylxanthines

Theophylline clearance is decreased by

- erythromycin
- cimetidine
- allopurinol
- frusemide
- oral contraceptives
- influenza vaccine

Aminophylline is an effective bronchodilator in acute asthma but it is no more effective than β stimulants and there are many more problems in its use. Therefore, it is best not used unless the response to nebulised β stimulants is inadequate. Toxic effects are common and occur with drug concentrations in or just above the therapeutic range. Concentrations are difficult to predict from the dose given because of individual differences in the rate of metabolism and interaction with drugs such as nicotine, cimetidine, and erythromycin.

Treatment of acute asthma

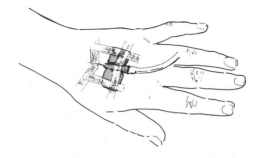

A loading injection of aminophylline must be given slowly over 15 minutes. When the patient is taking oral theophylline the dose should be reduced by at least 50%.

The position is further complicated when patients are already taking oral theophyllines. The usual starting dose for intravenous aminophylline is 5.6 mg/kg body weight given over 15 minutes. If the patient has taken oral theophylline or aminophylline in the previous 24 hours and a blood value is not available the initial dose should be halved. A continuous infusion is then given at a rate of 0.5 mg/kg/h, though this dose should be reduced if there is kidney or liver disease. If intravenous therapy is necessary for over 24 hours then blood concentrations will need to be determined (see chapter on Treatment of chronic asthma).

Corticosteroids

Side effects of a short course of corticosteroids

- Hyperglycaemia
- Hypokalaemia
- Fluid retention and hypertension
- Indigestion
- Mental changes
- Proximal myopathy
- Pancreatitis
- Glaucoma
- Gastrointestinal bleeding
- Allergic reactions to hydrocortisone
- Spread of infection

Uncommon

Corticosteroids are effective in preventing the development of acute severe asthma. Oral prednisolone should be given when control of asthma seems to be deteriorating in spite of adequate bronchodilator treatment. Twenty to 40 mg of prednisolone should be given in a single oral dose each day for seven to 14 days according to the speed of the response. The dose may then be tailed off slowly or, after short courses, stopped abruptly. If this opportunity is missed and acute asthma does develop corticosteroids are still very important. Fatal attacks of asthma are associated with failure to prescribe any or adequate doses of corticosteroids. No noticeable response occurs for four to six hours so it is important to begin corticosteroids early and to use intensive bronchodilator treatment while waiting for them to take effect.

In very severe asthma intravenous hydrocortisone should be used in an initial dose of 4 mg/kg body weight, followed by 3–4 mg/kg/6 h. After the first 24 hours if there has been a substantial improvement oral prednisolone should be substituted for hydrocortisone. Prednisolone should start at a dose of 40–60 mg/day and after the first dose hydrocortisone should be continued for six to 12 hours (50 mg prednisolone is equivalent to 200 mg hydrocortisone). If the patient is first seen at home and then transferred to hospital the first dose of corticosteroid should be given together with initial bronchodilator treatment before he leaves home. Less severe attacks can be managed throughout with oral rather than intravenous steroids.

The reduction in the dose of corticosteroids after an acute attack of asthma requiring hospital admission is governed by the patient's response. But it is important not to decrease the dose too quickly; and when intensive initial treatment has been required prednisolone should be maintained at 30 mg/day for at least one week. Two to three weeks' treatment may be needed to obtain the maximal response. There are few side effects of such short courses of corticosteroids.

Anticholinergic agents

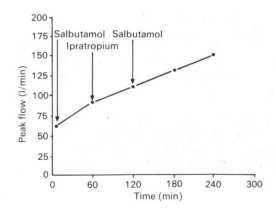

Ipratropium bromide has replaced atropine as the anticholinergic agent of choice in asthma as it has greater bronchial selectivity. Nebulised ipratropium appears to be as effective as a nebulised β stimulant in acute asthma. The dose of nebulised ipratropium is 500 μg or 1 mg, which should be diluted with saline rather than water. There are no problems with increased viscosity of secretions at this dose. Ipratropium has a slower onset of action than salbutamol: the peak response may not occur for 30 to 60 minutes. Adverse reactions such as paradoxical bronchoconstriction have occasionally been reported. These were mostly related to the osmolality of the solution or to preservatives. In the current preparations these have been corrected. β stimulants remain first line treatment, but nebulised ipratropium should be added if the response is not adequate. Some studies have shown a greater response to both drugs than to repeated β agonist alone and alternate nebulisations of the two drugs can be used at 60 to 120 minute intervals or the two drugs combined.

Antibiotics

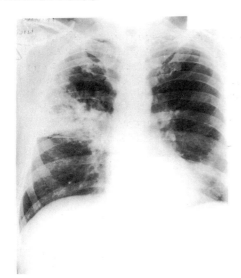

Upper respiratory tract infections are the commonest trigger factors for acute asthma.

Only in a few cases are acute exacerbations of asthma precipitated by bacterial infections. When respiratory infections are implicated they are usually caused by viruses. There is no evidence of benefit from the routine use of antibiotics, and these should be reserved for patients in whom there is presumptive evidence of infection such as fever, neutrophilia in blood or sputum, and radiological changes. In these circumstances, even though these features may occur in acute asthma without infection, an antibiotic such as amoxycillin or erythromycin should be included in the initial treatment.

Oxygen

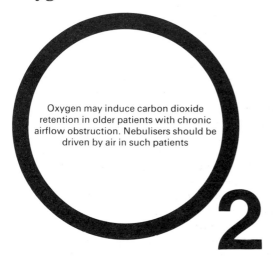

Oxygen may induce carbon dioxide retention in older patients with chronic airflow obstruction. Nebulisers should be driven by air in such patients

Acute severe asthma is always associated with hypoxia, although cyanosis develops late and is a grave sign. It is very unusual to provoke carbon dioxide retention with oxygen treatment in asthma, and oxygen should therefore be given freely during transfer to hospital, where blood gas measurements can be done. In older subjects with an exacerbation of chronic airflow obstruction and a potential danger of carbon dioxide retention initial treatment should be with 24% oxygen. Nebulisers should also be driven by oxygen rather than compressed air whenever possible, except in those with chronic airflow obstruction.

Fluid and electrolytes

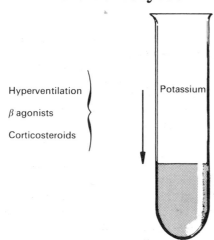

Hyperventilation

β agonists

Corticosteroids

Potassium

Patients with acute asthma tend to be depleted of fluid because they are often too breathless to drink and because fluid loss from the respiratory tract is increased. Dehydration increases the viscosity of mucus, increasing the likelihood of plugging in the airways. Intravenous fluid replacement is therefore often necessary in management. Three litres in the first 24 hours should be given if little oral fluid is being taken.

Hyperventilation, sympathomimetic drugs, and corticosteroids all tend to lower the serum potassium concentration. This is the most common electrolyte disturbance in acute asthma, and the serum potassium concentration should be monitored and supplements given as necessary.

Treatment of acute asthma

Controlled ventilation

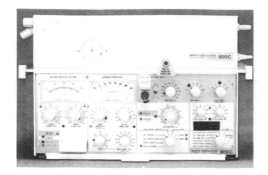

Occasionally mechanical ventilation is necessary for a short time while treatment takes effect. Usually it is necessary because the patient becomes exhausted, and experience and careful observation are necessary to judge the right time to begin this treatment. High inflation pressures and prolonged expiratory times may make ventilation difficult in asthmatic patients, but most experienced units have good results provided the decision to ventilate the patient is made electively and is not precipitated by a respiratory arrest. When mechanically ventilated patients fail to improve on adequate treatment bronchial lavage should be considered to reopen airways by removing plugs of mucus.

Other factors

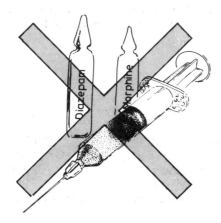

Most patients with acute severe asthma improve with these measures. Occasionally physiotherapy may be useful to help patients cough up thick sputum plugs, but mucolytic agents to change the nature of the secretions do not help.

An episode of severe asthma is frightening and the dangerous use of sedatives such as morphine was common before effective treatment became available. Unfortunately this practice still continues with occasional fatal consequences. Treatment of agitation should be aimed at reversing the asthma precipitating it, not at producing respiratory depression.

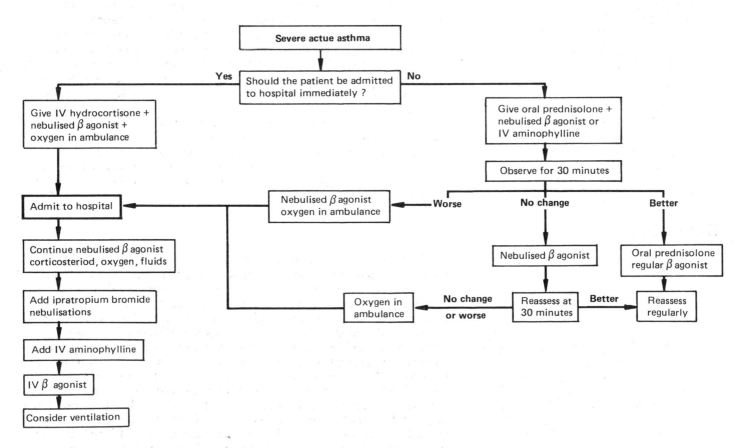

METHODS OF DRUG DELIVERY

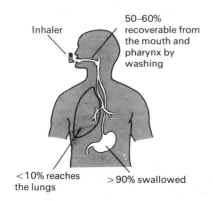

Inhaler

50–60% recoverable from the mouth and pharynx by washing

<10% reaches the lungs

>90% swallowed

Various devices and formulations have been developed that deliver drugs efficiently, minimise side effects, and are easy to use. With the range of devices now available it is possible for most patients to use inhalers. In some circumstances oral therapy is needed and the methods of producing sustained oral release have also become much more sophisticated.

Metered dose inhalers

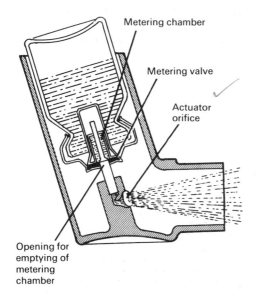

Metering chamber

Metering valve

Actuator orifice

Opening for emptying of metering chamber

Inhalers deliver the drug directly to the airways. A metered dose inhaler deposits just under 10% of the drug into the airways beyond the larynx. Nearly all the rest of the dose impacts in the oropharynx and is swallowed. This swallowed portion may be absorbed from the gastrointestinal tract, but drugs such as inhaled corticosteroids are almost completely removed by first pass metabolism in the liver.

An important point in the prescription of inhalation therapy is to instruct the patient in the technique. He should start the inhaler mechanism immediately after beginning to breathe in slowly and deeply, then hold his breath for 10 seconds. The technique should be checked periodically. About 25% of patients have difficulty in using a metered dose inhaler. Some arthritic patients find it hard to exert enough downward pressure to start an inhaler; they can be helped by a "Haleraid" device, which responds to squeezing.

Breath actuated inhalers are available for β agonist therapy. The valve of the inhaler is actuated as the patient breathes in. The new devices respond to a quite low inspiratory airflow and can be useful for those who have difficulty in coordinating actuation and breathing. The inhaler clicks and vibrates when it begins to operate; this can interrupt inspiration in some patients.

Extension tubes

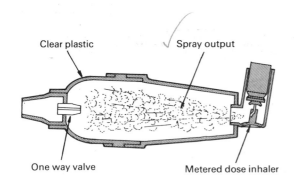

Clear plastic

Spray output

One way valve

Metered dose inhaler

The coordination of aerosol firing and inspiration becomes slightly less important when a short extension tube is used; this may help if problems are minor. A 0.75 litre reservoir removes all need for coordination of breathing and actuation. The inhaler is fixed into the chamber and the breath is taken from a one way valve at the other end of the chamber. A little over 10% of the drug reaches the airways. Pharyngeal deposition is greatly reduced since the faster particles impact in the chamber, not the mouth, and evaporation of propellant from the slower particles produces a small sized aerosol, which penetrates better into the lungs. This is particularly useful for the minority of patients who develop oral candidiasis with inhaled corticosteroid therapy. The device is cumbersome; but this is no great disadvantage for corticosteroid therapy, which usually needs to be carried out only twice a day. These chambers can be used for all types of inhalers and have proved useful in acute asthma. But they have no advantage for patients who can use a metered dose inhaler effectively and have no problems with oral thrush.

Methods of drug delivery
Dry powder inhalers ✓

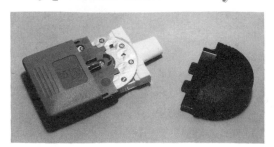

Dry powder inhalers of various types are available for β agonists, sodium cromoglycate, and corticosteroids. Since inspiratory airflow releases the fine powder, problems of breath coordination are avoided. Worries about the environmental consequences of aerosol propellants are also avoided. The dry powder makes some patients cough. The inconvenience of reloading for each administration has been overcome in the newer multidose devices, which contain 8 or 200 doses.

Nebulisers

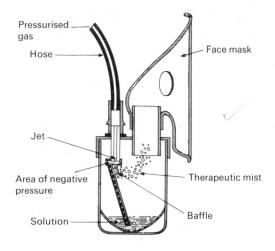

Nebulisers can be driven by compressed gas or an ultrasonically vibrating crystal. They provide a way of administering inhaled drugs to those unable to use any other device. This may be the case in the very young or in acute attacks, when inspiratory airflow is limited. Nebulisers also offer a convenient way of delivering a higher dose to the airways. About 12% of the drug leaving the chamber enters the lungs, but most of the dose stays in the apparatus or is wasted in expiration. Delivery depends on the type of nebuliser, the flow rate at which it is driven, and the volume in the chamber. In most cases flow rates below 6 or 8 l/min give too large a particle size and nebulise too slowly. Newer chambers have a reservoir and valve system to reduce loss during expiration.

Parenteral administration

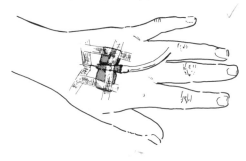

Injections are usually used only for the treatment of acute attacks. Subcutaneous injections may be useful in emergencies when nebuliser apparatus is unavailable. Occasional patients with severe chronic asthma seem to benefit from the high levels of β stimulant obtained with continuous subcutaneous infusion from a battery driven pump.

A loading injection of aminophylline must be given slowly over 15 minutes. When the patient is taking oral theophylline the dose should be reduced by at least 50%.

Oral

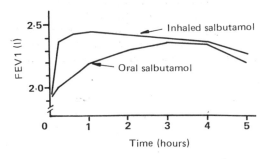

Tablets and syrups are available for oral use. This route is necessary for theophyllines, which cannot be inhaled effectively. Children who are unable to inhale drugs can take the sugar free liquid preparations. Slow release tablets are used when a prolonged action is needed, particularly for nocturnal asthma (p 3), where theophyllines and β agonists have proved helpful. Various slow release mechanisms have been developed to maintain even blood levels. These include a tablet coating pierced by a laser drilled hole through which salbutamol is slowly released.

TREATMENT OF CHRONIC ASTHMA

β Stimulants

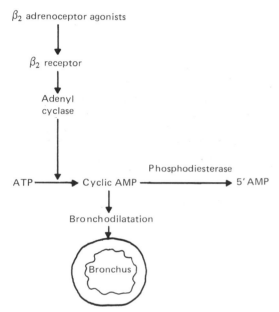

β_2 adrenoceptor agonists

β_2 receptor

Adenyl cyclase

ATP ⟶ Cyclic AMP ⟶ 5' AMP

Phosphodiesterase

Bronchodilatation

Bronchus

The mainstay of treatment of mild intermittent asthma is one of the selective β_2 stimulants taken by inhalation. Their onset of action is fast, and salbutamol, terbutaline, and fenoterol have an effect lasting for four to six hours. If more than occasional doses are required their regular use should be considered, with additional symptomatic use as necessary. It makes little sense rigidly to restrict the daily dose to two puffs four times a day when an initial nebuliser dose in hospital may be five to 10 times this total dose. The dose needed varies between patients, as does the dose producing side effects such as tremor. A maximum daily dose, perhaps 20 puffs, should be established so that the patient can seek help if he feels he needs to exceed this threshold dose. Patients should be taught to monitor their inhaler use and to understand that if this increases or its effects get less these are danger signals. They indicate deterioration in asthmatic control and suggest the need for further treatment.

Some studies have suggested that β stimulants may become slightly less effective with continued use, particularly if the dose is high; others have failed to find evidence of this tachyphylaxis. But in all studies it has been found to be a minor effect quickly reversed by temporarily stopping the therapy or by corticosteroid treatment.

β agonists have a wide safety margin. Tremor, palpitations, and muscle cramps may occur but are rarely troublesome if the drug is inhaled.

Anticholinergic bronchodilators

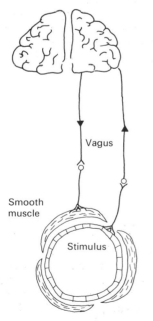

Vagus

Smooth muscle

Stimulus

Ipratropium bromide blocks the cholinergic bronchoconstrictor effect of the vagus nerve. It is the only anticholinergic agent widely available for inhaled use and is most effective in very young children and older patients. In young asthmatic patients it is in most cases less effective than β stimulants but it may supplement their effect when reversibility is incomplete. Ipratropium bromide takes second place as a bronchodilator in asthma unless tremor is troublesome with β stimulants. If the response to a β stimulant is inadequate then the technique of using the inhaler should be checked first. If this is satisfactory evidence of an extra anticholinergic effect should be sought by measuring peak flow before and after the β agonist and then 30–60 minutes after adding ipratropium. At these doses drying of secretions or interference with mucociliary clearance does not occur.

Anticholinergic agents block vagal efferent stimulation of bronchial smooth muscle.

Treatment of chronic asthma
Methylxanthines

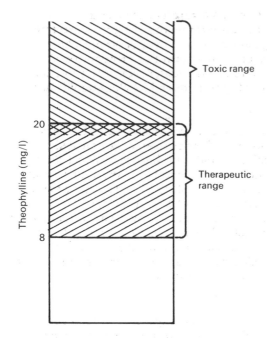

There is no safety margin between therapeutic and toxic ranges with theophylline.

Theophylline has often been used as a first line agent for asthma in North America. Its safety margin is low, however, and individual differences in the doses required are high, so that treatment is best monitored by measuring blood concentrations. Inhaled treatment with β agonists is much preferable, but some patients who respond to β agonists benefit from added theophylline, especially for symptoms at night. In these cases a slow release oral preparation containing theophylline or its ethylene diamine salt, aminophylline, should be used. Absorption of aminophylline from suppositories is much less predictable and they are best avoided.

The commonest side effects of theophylline are nausea, vomiting, and abdominal discomfort, but headache, malaise, fast pulse rates, and fits also occur, sometimes without warning from gastrointestinal symptoms. The dose of theophylline should start at around 7 mg/kg/day, in divided doses, doubling if no response occurs. If any side effects occur or if the dose rises above twice this starting dose the blood concentrations of theophylline must be measured. Ideally all patients taking theophylline should have their concentrations monitored and doses adjusted until there are between 10 and 20 mg/l (50–100 μmol/l). Above 20 mg/l toxic effects are unacceptably high, although 15–30% of patients will have gastrointestinal effects below this level. Theophylline clearance is increased by smoking, alcohol consumption, and enzyme inducing drugs such as phenytoin, rifampicin, and barbiturates. Clearance will be decreased and blood levels rise with cimetidine or erythromycin treatment and in the presence of heart failure, liver impairment, and pneumonia.

Sodium cromoglycate and nedocromil sodium

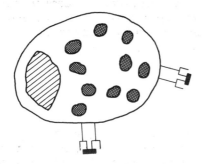

Mast cell

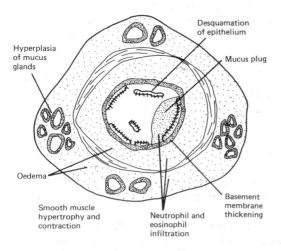

The pathological changes in the airway in asthma. Airway inflammation persists even in remission.

Sodium cromoglycate is able to block bronchoconstrictor responses to challenge by exercise and antigens. The conventionally accepted mechanism of mast cell stabilisation is currently under question as the main mechanism of its action in asthma. It is used as the first line prophylactic agent after failure to control asthma with occasional inhalation of a β agonist. Success is most likely with young atopic asthmatics but may occur at all ages. Sodium cromoglycate was usually given as plain spincaps containing 20 mg of the drug as a dry powder, but metered dose inhalers delivering 5 mg per inhalation are also available and are more convenient and just as effective. Occasionally patients develop reflex bronchoconstriction in response to the irritant effects of the dry powder. This problem can be treated by giving a β agonist just before, by switching to the metered dose inhaler, or by giving compound spincaps containing 0.1 mg isoprenaline in addition to the 20 mg of cromoglycate. The last alternative is the least satisfactory as patients recognise the immediate bronchodilator effect of the isoprenaline and then tend to use the preparation inappropriately.

Other adverse reactions to sodium cromoglycate are rare, and this helps to explain the resistance to oral alternatives such as ketotifen, which produces drowsiness in about 10% of patients. Cromoglycate should not be dismissed as ineffective until it has been tried for at least four weeks, and its use must be regular. It has no place in acute exacerbations of asthma and may even increase narrowing of the airways by its irritant effect.

Nedocromil sodium has the same properties as sodium cromoglycate but may have an additional anti-inflammatory effect on the airway epithelium. It is probably more useful than sodium cromoglycate in older patients although less effective than inhaled corticosteroids in most cases.

Corticosteroids

Many acute episodes of asthma are preceded by a period of poor control. Most patients can be taught to detect this deterioration and prevent a severe attack by starting themselves on a short course of oral corticosteroids

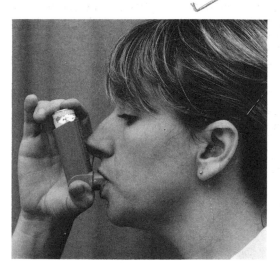

The dose of inhaled corticosteroid should be adjusted for each patient. Clinically important adrenal suppression does not occur below 1500 μg/day of beclomethasone dipropionate (or its equivalent).

Occasional asthmatic patients end up taking long term oral corticosteroids but this should be only after failure of vigorous treatment with other drugs, and the symptoms or risks of the disease must be balanced against the adverse effects of long term treatment with oral corticosteroids. It is important to remember that, in contrast, short courses of oral steroids for exacerbations of symptoms and inhaled steroids have few problems.

Inhaled steroids are given by metered dose inhaler or one of the other inhalation devices used for β agonists. The dose should be adjusted to produce optimum control. Inhaled steroids may be given twice daily with no problems apart from occasional oropharyngeal candidiasis or a husky voice until a daily dose above the equivalent of 1500 μg beclomethasone dipropionate is reached. At higher doses biochemical evidence of suppression of the hypothalamic–pituitary–adrenal axis may be found even with inhaled steroids, but this is not a clinical problem in adults. Inhaled steroids must be taken regularly to be effective and have no place in treating acute asthma. Once inhaled steroids are being taken there seems to be no benefit to be gained from adding or continuing sodium cromoglycate.

Short courses of steroids may be stopped abruptly or tailed off over a few days. Low cortisol and ACTH concentrations are found for two to three days after 40 mg prednisolone for three weeks, but clinical problems with responses to stress or exacerbations of asthma seem not to occur. A typical course would be 30–40 mg prednisolone for 14 days. Most asthmatic patients can be taught to keep such a supply of steroids at home and use them when predetermined signs of deteriorating control occur. If patients require long term oral corticosteroids, they should be stabilised on an alternate day regimen whenever possible, the goal always remaining to discontinue long term steroids in the future. They should be combined with inhaled steroids in moderately high doses to keep the dose of oral steroids as low as possible. Alternative preparations such as triamcinolone and ACTH are less flexible to use than prednisolone and have no advantages in terms of adrenal suppression.

Desensitisation and allergen avoidance

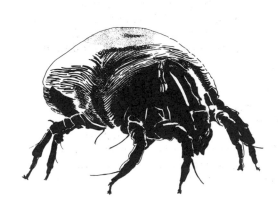

As discussed in the chapter on Precipitating factors, the results of trials of desensitisation and allergen avoidance have been disappointing. Some patients have obvious precipitating factors—in particular, animals—and avoidance is helpful but usually leaves other unknown precipitating factors. More common are patients with reactive airways and sensitivity to pollens, house dust mites, and other allergens. Such stimuli are almost impossible to avoid in everyday life, although symptoms improve with rigorous measures such as admission to a dust free environment in hospital.

There is some evidence that desensitisation is beneficial in pollen asthma and that repeated courses increase the improvement. Controlled studies in adults sensitive to house dust mites have shown no benefit from desensitisation. Several studies in children have suggested some benefit, but these were all highly selected patients, and it is unusual to find asthmatic patients with a single sensitivity. The degree of control produced by desensitisation can usually be achieved with simple, safe inhaled therapy.

There is no sound evidence to support desensitisation to other agents in asthmatic patients. In particular, cocktails produced from the results of skin tests or radioallergosorbent tests are not a valid form of treatment. Local reactions to desensitising infections are common and more generalised reactions and even deaths occur. Most deaths are related to mistakes in the injection schedule. Courses of injections should only be given where appropriate facilities for resuscitation are available.

Combination therapy and other treatments

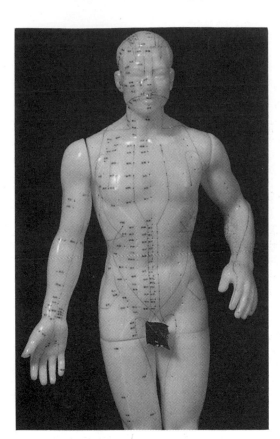

In a variable disease such as asthma where treatment should be regularly tailored to the state of the disease it seems particularly illogical to use fixed dose combinations. Several such oral preparations are still available, often containing small doses of theophylline, ephedrine, and a barbiturate. Although some patients with mild asthma exist happily taking such preparations, there is no indication for prescribing them to new patients. Some inhaled combination preparations are available but these also restrict the flexibility of treatment. Combinations of corticosteroid and β stimulant can lead to inappropirate use. Mixtures of β stimulant and anticholinergic may be useful when the combination of these two bronchodilators has been found to be appropriate.

Other drugs such as α stimulants, antihistamines, and calcium antagonists have occasionally been found to have some effect. Nevertheless, they have no great practical value in asthma.

There have been dramatic claims for the benefit of yoga, hypnosis, and acupuncture but few have been confirmed in controlled trials. Relaxation may help to reduce anxiety and hyperventilation, which can exacerbate asthma. Ionisation of inspired air may produce a small effect on lung function and may attenuate the response to exercise, but such effects are minimal and not achieved by home ionisers. Herbal remedies may contain conventional agents but are not usually standardised; some have even been found to contain corticosteroids.

Many oral and inhaled combined preparations are available, but in a variable disease such as asthma they can produce confusion and difficulties in obtaining the necessary flexibility of treatment

ASTHMA IN CHILDREN: DIAGNOSIS AND ASSESSMENT

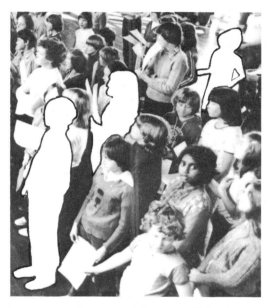

In an average primary school class three children have asthma: two boys, one girl.

Asthma is one of the commonest causes of ill health in childhood. More absence from school is due to asthma than to any other chronic condition; 30% of asthmatic children miss more than three weeks of schooling each year. Over the past 20 years there has been a steady increase in the reported prevalence of childhood asthma in the United Kingdom and in the number of general practice consultations and hospital admissions. More recently there has been an increase in asthma deaths. Despite a greater awareness of the condition by doctors and parents, there remains the problem of definition, especially in the very young, and the diagnosis of asthma is often delayed or not made.

At least 11% of schoolchildren suffer from recurrent attacks of wheezing. Asthma is more common in boys than in girls (2:1), and boys tend to have more severe symptoms. After puberty this sex difference disappears. About 80% of asthmatic children develop symptoms before the age of 5 years and a third before the age of 2 years. Fortunately the mortality is low but 40 to 50 children die of asthma each year in England and Wales.

The clinical presentation, response to treatment, and prognosis differ in important ways from those in adults, and the fact that the patient is a child poses special problems. When planning management one should not merely extrapolate from experience with adult asthma.

Bronchial reactivity and allergy

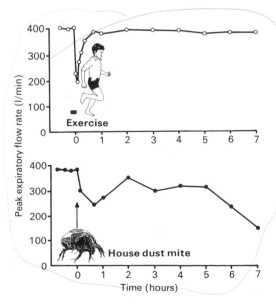

Airway obstruction induced by exercise and allergy in an asthmatic child. In severe asthma the late (4–8 hour) reaction to allergen may be important.

Increased bronchial reactivity is a major feature of childhood asthma and nearly all asthmatic children with symptoms severe enough to warrant hospital referral give immediate allergic skin reactions to environmental antigens. Recent studies have confirmed, however, that some asthmatic children do not demonstrate increased bronchial reactivity in laboratory tests and some have no evidence of "atopic" allergy. Conversely, there are children with no respiratory symptoms, despite demonstrable bronchial hyperreactivity, and many children with positive skin tests have no clinical evidence that the allergens to which they react in the skin provoke attacks of asthma. It is important not to rely entirely on tests for these characteristics when considering the diagnosis of asthma in a child.

Ninety per cent of asthmatic children show increased bronchial sensitivity to inhaled histamine; three quarters develop bronchial obstruction during a standardised exercise test and exercise will provoke wheezing in nearly all children with moderate or severe asthma. Bronchial responsiveness is to some extent genetically controlled, but there are also important environmental inducers of airway hyperresponsiveness. In children the most important of these are viral respiratory infections and exposure to certain allergens.

The importance of allergy in childhood asthma is sometimes overstressed: allergic reactions are rarely the sole cause of a child's wheezing. Over 80% of asthmatic children become sensitised at some time to the house dust mite and about 60% to pollens and animal danders.

Asthma in children: diagnosis and assessment

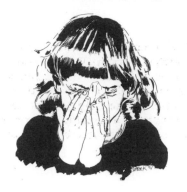

Rather fewer preschool children with asthma are atopic; about three quarters of those with frequent wheezing have positive skin tests and elevated serum levels of IgE. Children with perennial asthma often show a dual response to experimental inhalation of allergen; a short lasting and easily reversible immediate response is followed by a more severe and protracted late response. The late response is still not understood but it leads to an increase in bronchial reactivity and may be important in children with severe symptoms.

Young children who wheeze only in association with viral respiratory infections (recurrent "wheezy bronchitis") show the same characteristics of bronchial reactivity and allergy. They have, and should be treated as having, mild asthma.

The wheezy infant

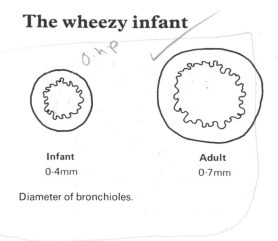

Infant
0·4mm

Adult
0·7mm

Diameter of bronchioles.

"Fat happy wheezers"

Post-bronchiolitis wheezers

Atopic wheezers

Wheezing is a very common symptom in the first year of life and there are good reasons why infants are prone to airways obstruction. Their bronchi are narrower and have less rigid walls than those of older children, and a baby's compliant chest wall allows the airways to collapse towards the end of expiration. In the past it was thought that infants' airways might be deficient in smooth muscle and beta adrenergic receptors. We now know that wheezy infants have both smooth muscle and effective beta adrenoreceptors in their intrathoracic airways because they show a bronchoconstrictor response to histamine or nebulised water which can be prevented with nebulised salbutamol.

Many babies have recurrent episodes of loud wheezing and mild tachypnoea, apparently associated with viral respiratory tract infections, but they remain well and gain weight normally; indeed they may be overweight. Recurrent cough and wheezing frequently follow acute viral bronchiolitis. About 1% of babies are admitted to hospital with this infection which is usually caused by the respiratory syncitial virus (RSV). In later childhood these children have abnormal airways lability, although most stop wheezing before they go to school. A personal or family history of "atopic" disease is no more prevalent than in the general population; this suggests that the RSV infection causes abnormal bronchial reactivity in children otherwise not especially predisposed to asthma. A third group of wheezy babies have eczema and/or a strong family history of asthma, eczema, or hay fever. They are more likely than the other two groups to have asthma which persists throughout childhood.

Diagnosis

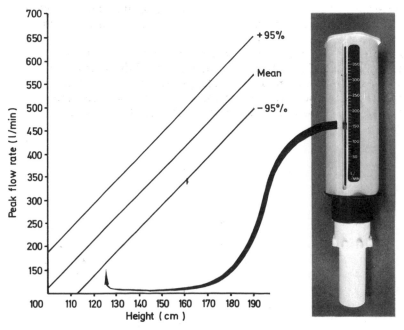

Peak flow rate (l/min) vs Height (cm). Curves labelled +95%, Mean, −95%.

At least 90% of recurrent wheezing in childhood is due to asthma and in most cases the diagnosis can be made from a carefully taken history after explaining what is meant by a wheeze. Some 15–20% of asthmatic children develop symptoms before they are a year old and 80% before they are 5 years. A low reading peak flow meter is available for use in young children and the results can be related to established normal values. If the peak flow is lower than expected asthma can be confirmed by a rise of at least 20% after a bronchodilator. Absence of wheeze or a normal peak flow reading at one examination does not of course exclude asthma, and it may be helpful to do a simple running exercise test to see whether this induces bronchoconstriction. Skin tests and measurement of total and specific IgE will only establish whether the child is atopic and a chest radiograph is done more to look for other causes of wheezing than to diagnose asthma.

Causes of wheezing in children

- Asthma
- Bronchiolitis
- Inhalation:
  foreign body
  milk
- Cystic fibrosis
- Tuberculosis
- Bronchomalacia
- Tracheal or bronchial stenosis
- Vascular rings
- Mediastinal masses

Young children sometimes present with recurrent cough but apparently no wheezing or breathlessness. The cough is worse at night and often associated with viral respiratory infections or exercise. If the child is too young to use a peak flow meter a therapeutic trial of a bronchodilator given regularly may be helpful. If the cough resolves the child has asthma.

Providing that the diagnosis leads to appropriate treatment parents' anxiety is much more likely to be relieved than increased by being told that their child has asthma.

Patterns of illness

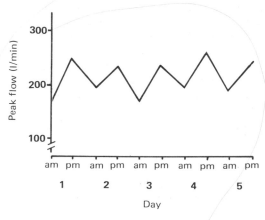

Poorly controlled asthma.

It is important to establish the frequency and severity of the asthma and what triggers wheezing; also whether the child is missing school, whether he is able to take part in normal sport, and the impact on the rest of the family. Chest deformity indicates chronic airways obstruction; growth retardation is only seen when a child has severe continuous symptoms. Lung function can be assessed over a period by recording the peak flow rate twice daily at home. If the peak flow is consistently lower than expected or shows wide variation the child's asthma is poorly controlled. More sensitive tests of airway obstruction or measurements of lung volume are valuable when assessing lung function between attacks. Skin tests and measurement of serum IgE antibodies may be a useful adjunct to the history but should not be overinterpreted.

Asthmatic children can roughly be divided into three groups, which provide a useful guide to management.

About three quarters have infrequent acute episodes of wheezing, usually associated with signs of viral upper respiratory infection. The episodes vary in duration and in some cases are quite severe but lung function returns completely to normal between attacks. Eighty per cent of these children will stop wheezing before adulthood.

About a quarter have more frequent and prolonged wheezing triggered by infective, allergic, emotional, and physical stimuli. Their asthma often starts with similar symptoms to those of the first group but at a younger age. In most of these children sensitive indices of airflow obstruction are abnormal between attacks, though the peak flow may return to normal.

A third, small group have severe wheezing which continues throughout childhood. Four out of 5 are boys, symptoms start before the age of 2, and many also have eczema and rhinitis. There is usually a strong family history of atopy. These children tend to be small and thin and to develop chest deformities. All have abnormal lung function between attacks and most continue to wheeze as adults.

A few, generally older children with grass pollen allergy, wheeze predominantly from May to July. Most asthmatic children, however, have more trouble in the winter months. This is probably because viral respiratory tract infections are more common in winter and because exercise induced asthma is more likely to develop outdoors in cold weather.

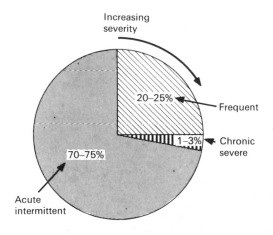

ASTHMA IN CHILDREN: TREATMENT

Drug treatment at home

Management of childhood asthma at home	
Symptoms	*Drugs*
Intermittent, associated mainly with respiratory infections	Intermittent: salbutamol, terbutaline, or ipratropium bromide
Frequent, triggered by infection, allergy, exercise, physical and emotional factors	Continuous: cromoglycate or theophylline + Intermittent: bronchodilators
Failure to respond to above or severe persistent wheezing	Continuous: beclomethasone or budesonide + bronchodilators ± theophylline

Chest deformity like this is an indication to treat with inhaled steroids.

Drugs, when taken properly, are very effective in most asthmatic children, but much depends on the family and there are several booklets which help with explanation. The choice of drugs depends on the overall severity of the asthma. As the child grows older asthma may improve or become worse, so treatment needs to be reviewed regularly.

Children with episodic asthma need only intermittent treatment with bronchodilators, though they may have to take a bronchodilator regularly during and for a week or two after a viral respiratory infection. Over the age of 2 beta adrenergic agonists are more effective than anticholinergic agents. Inhaled drugs act faster than oral ones and the inhaled dose is smaller, so the risk of side effects is less. Although drugs taken by mouth act relatively slowly they have a place in the treatment of patients who are unable to use inhalers—for example, the very young or those who are handicapped.

Children with frequent asthma need drugs which prevent wheezing. Indications for prescribing a prophylactic agent are symptoms on most days, at least one asthma attack per month, and failure of lung function to return to normal between attacks. Chest deformity, with bowing forward of the sternum and "Harrison's sulci," is an absolute indication for prophylaxis.

The prophylactic drugs are sodium cromoglycate, slow or controlled release oral bronchodilators, ketotifen, and inhaled steroids. Regular, four times daily sodium cromoglycate powder controls symptoms in 50–60% of children with frequent asthma. It is safe but the need for frequent administration is inconvenient, especially when the inhaler has to be taken to school. Cromoglycate solution via a nebuliser improves symptoms in preschool asthma but fails to reduce the hospital admission rate.

Slow release oral theophylline preparations given twice daily, in doses titrated to maintain blood levels of 10–20 mg/l, have a similar efficacy to cromoglycate. There is no advantage in giving both drugs together. The problems with theophylline treatment are a wide individual variation in clearance rates and a high incidence of side effects.

Children need larger doses of theophylline relative to body weight than adults. Theophylline clearance is retarded during viral infections, when toxic levels may occur, and by some commonly used drugs—for example, erythromycin. Gastrointestinal side effects and behavioural problems are frequent even when blood levels are within the "therapeutic range" and theophyllines may affect sleep patterns. A single dose of a slow release theophylline taken at bedtime will reduce nocturnal asthma. Nocturnal cough and wheezing are often an indication of poor overall asthma control and inhaled cromoglycate or steroids taken regularly during the day will also improve symptoms at night. Preliminary trials with a controlled release salbutamol preparation suggest it has a similar therapeutic effect to slow release theophylline in therapeutic concentrations but has a lower incidence of adverse reactions.

Ketotifen is an antihistamine with antianaphylactic properties. The results of the early low dose clinical trials were disappointing. Subsequent trials using higher doses and longer treatment periods have shown some benefit in mild and seasonal asthma but have failed to demonstrate any therapeutic effect on young children with frequent asthma.

Inhaled corticosteroids given twice daily by metered dose aerosol or by dry powder inhaler are more powerful prophylactic agents than either cromoglycate or controlled release bronchodilators. In preschool children

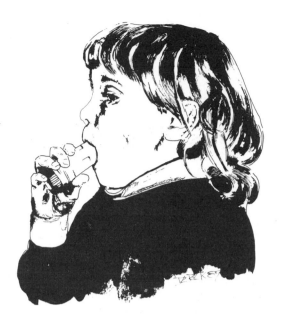

nebulised beclomethasone solution is relatively ineffective, but this is probably because it is difficult to deliver adequate doses of the rather insoluble beclomethasone through the nebuliser. Budesonide inhaled through a Nebuhaler significantly improves asthma in 2–6 year olds with frequent perennial symptoms. Although there is biochemical evidence of adrenal suppression in some children receiving inhaled steroids, long term administration has not been shown to cause clinically significant systemic effects. Cromoglycate combined with an inhaled steroid is no better than the inhaled steroid alone, but children with severe asthma which is not fully controlled with inhaled steroids benefit from the concurrent use of either a beta agonist or theophylline. Children taking prophylactic drugs should always have available a fast acting bronchodilator to treat acute attacks.

Because of the risk of side effects and the availability of inhaled steroids, long term treatment with oral steroids should only be used in children with serious asthma which cannot be controlled in other ways; a single dose should be given on alternate days whenever possible. Recent trials have shown that a short course or even a single large dose of prednisolone speeds recovery from an acute asthma attack. The need for short courses of oral steroids is, however, an indication to review the overall management of a child's asthma.

Inhalers

Inhalers used to treat children with asthma under the age of 10 years.

Age (years)	Inhaler device	Treatment Bronchodilator	Prophylaxis
Under 2	nebuliser	ipratropium bromide salbutamol terbutaline	cromoglycate
2–4	nebuliser	salbutamol terbutaline	cromoglycate beclomethasone budesonide
	Nebuhaler	terbutaline	budesonide ?cromoglycate
	Volumatic	salbutamol	?beclomethasone
4–10	*As above plus*		
	Rotahaler/ Diskhaler	salbutamol	beclomethasone
	Turbohaler	terbutaline	—
	Spinhaler	—	cromoglycate
	Aerolin Auto	salbutamol	—
	Spacer Inhaler	terbutaline	budesonide

The most common reasons for failure of inhaled treatment in asthmatic children are the use of inappropriate inhalers or the incorrect use of appropriate inhalers. Children become fully aware of their own breathing and recognise the difference between inspiration and expiration by about the age of 3 years. Until then the only useful inhalation devices are those which can be applied during tidal breathing. Even when a child can manage a controlled deep inspiration, inspiratory flow rates are slower and airway diameters are smaller than in adults and this may influence the site of deposition of the drug particles. Few children under the age of 10 years can manage unmodified metered dose aerosols. Those who master the technique when they are well often find they cannot do it when they are breathless and wheezing. The choice of inhaler device depends on the child's age; the child's and the family's preference for a particular inhaler is also important.

Nebulisers are not available on prescription but many are being sold for home use. Asthma prophylaxis can be given to young children by nebuliser and hospital admission may sometimes be avoided by prompt administration of high dose nebulised bronchodilator at home. Main concerns about home nebulisers are lack of proper instruction in their use and delay in seeking medical advice during a severe asthma attack. Another worry is that, in both infants and older children, administration of a nebulised bronchodilator may lead to a fall in oxygenation. This effect could be enhanced if, as sometimes happens in severe asthma, there is no improvement in the airways obstruction after the bronchodilator. Nevertheless, there is an important place for the judicious use of home nebulisers in young asthmatic children.

Antigen avoidance and hyposensitisation

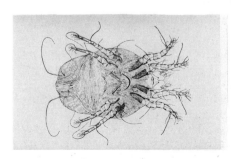

Measures taken to eradicate the house dust mite, *D pteronyssinus*, from the bedrooms of asthmatic children who are sensitised might be expected to improve nocturnal symptoms. The results of controlled trials have been disappointing, perhaps because the most stringent measures only incompletely or transiently remove the mites. Certain acaride sprays reduce the levels of *D pteronyssinus* for long periods after a single application; it remains to be seen whether they are of clinical value. Families with an asthmatic child should be encouraged not to acquire pet animals. The removal of household pets is more contentious unless there is a clear history of sensitivity, because the emotional upset may make things

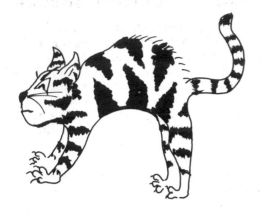

worse. The relationship of food and drink to asthma is not well understood and there is a poor correlation between the history and challenge tests in the laboratory. Nevertheless, certain dietary allergens (milk, eggs, nuts), chemicals (tartrazine), and physical agents (ice) may increase bronchial reactivity in some children with asthma.

In carefully selected asthmatic children hyposensitisation with house dust mite, cat, dog, and mould antigen results in a modest clinical improvement. The evidence of benefit from pollen hyposensitisation in children with asthma is inconclusive. The treatment is painful, expensive, time consuming, and occasionally dangerous. When one considers that most childhood asthma is provoked by non-allergenic as well as by specific allergic triggers and that drug therapy is very safe there seems little justification for resorting to hyposensitisation therapy.

Asthma in infancy

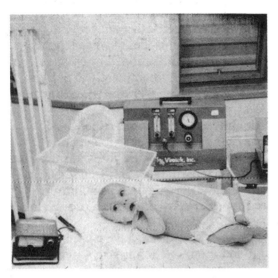

A baby with persistent wheezing dating from soon after birth may need investigation for rare causes. Very few wheezy infants will gain measurable benefit from bronchodilator drugs. The reason for this is unknown. Babies who wheeze when they have viral respiratory infections but are otherwise well ("fat happy wheezers") are unlikely to respond to any asthma drug and the most important aspect of management is reassurance and observation to ensure that they continue to thrive. It is certainly worth trying beta adrenergic stimulants on those who have troublesome wheezing, particularly if they have eczema or a strong family history of asthma ("atopic wheezers"). A rather larger proportion of wheezy infants seem to respond to nebulised ipratropium bromide. The response is unpredictable and the only way to find out which babies will benefit is by a therapeutic trial. The little information available about oral theophylline suggests it is no more effective than beta agonists in relieving bronchoconstriction during infancy. Difficulties with administration and the poor results from clinical studies do not justify the use of nebulised cromoglycate or the currently available nebulisable steroids in babies under one year. Controlled trials have failed to show any benefit from systemic steroids at this age. Acute severe wheezing is best managed in hospital, where the mainstay of treatment is hydration and oxygen and where the response to beta stimulants and ipratropium bromide can be assessed.

Acute severe asthma

Some indications for hospital admission	
Signs	cyanosis exhaustion difficulty speaking pulsus paradoxus > 20 mm
PEFR	< 25% of predicted
Response	no improvement despite adequate doses of inhaled bronchodilator
Experience	known pattern of attacks

Parents and children need clear instructions on what to do when an acute asthma attack occurs and when to ask for medical help. If the attack does not respond quickly to the child's usual relief medication treatment should be given with a large dose of a beta stimulant bronchodilator (salbutamol, terbutaline) by nebuliser or Nebuhaler. Subcutaneous terbutaline 0.005 mg (0.01 ml)/kg is less satisfactory because of distress caused by the injection. Consideration should be given to starting oral prednisolone. The response to treatment should be documented objectively in all children old enough to use a peak flow meter. A child who responds well to a high dose of nebulised bronchodilator at home will need to be reviewed a few hours later, and will require increased treatment for a week or more afterwards.

The principles of assessment and treatment in hospital of children over the age of 18 months are similar to those in adults, though some children recover without the need for systemic steroids. When faced with an intravenous infusion young children sometimes become very distressed and make their asthma worse, in which case it may be better to treat them with nebulised salbutamol and ipratropium bromide and oral steroids.

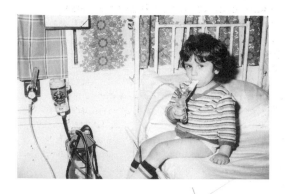

Oxygen is important in treatment but sometimes difficult to give to toddlers. Dehydration occurs because of poor fluid intake, sweating, and, in the early stages, hyperventilation. This must be corrected, but there are potential risks in overhydrating children with severe asthma. Production of antidiuretic hormone may be increased during the attack, and the considerable negative intrathoracic pressures generated by the respiratory efforts may predispose to pulmonary oedema. After correcting dehydration the wisest course is to give normal fluid requirements and measure the plasma and urine osmolality.

A child should not be discharged from hospital until he is taking the treatment he will be taking at home, and on this treatment the peak flow rate should be at least 75% of expected.

Management of severe asthma in hospital

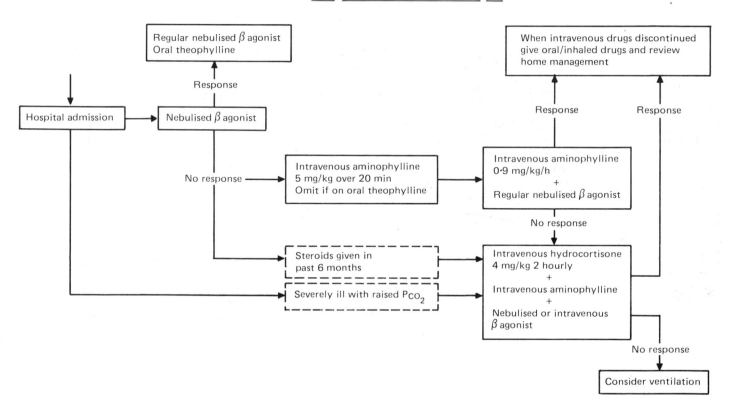

INDEX

Index